D1609340

THE ⊗ FILES™

1997 desk diary

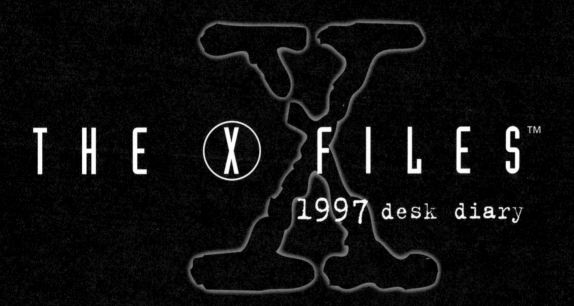

THE ⊗ FILES™

1997 desk diary

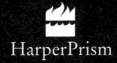

HarperPrism

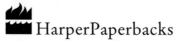 HarperPaperbacks
A Division of HarperCollins*Publishers*
10 East 53rd Street, New York, N.Y. 10022-5299

We wish to acknowledge the following still photographers for their photographic contributions to this book:
Michael Grecco
Chris Helcermanas-Benge
Jack Rowand
Ken Staniforth
Marcel Williams

 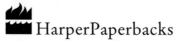
HarperPaperbacks may be purchased for educational, business, or sales promotional use. For information, please write:
Special Markets Department, HarperCollins*Publishers,*
10 East 53rd Street, New York, N.Y. 10022-5299.

Printed in the United States of America

First printing: August 1996

Designed by Derek Walls
Research assistance by Sarah Stegall

Visit HarperPaperbacks on the World Wide Web at
http://www.harpercollins.com/paperbacks

96 97 98 99 ❖ 10 9 8 7 6 5 4 3 2 1

THE Ⓧ FILES™
1997 desk diary

1997

january
s	m	t	w	t	f	s
			1	2	3	4
5	6	7	8	9	10	11
12	13	14	15	16	17	18
19	20	21	22	23	24	25
26	27	28	29	30	31	

february
s	m	t	w	t	f	s
						1
2	3	4	5	6	7	8
9	10	11	12	13	14	15
16	17	18	19	20	21	22
23	24	25	26	27	28	

march
s	m	t	w	t	f	s
						1
2	3	4	5	6	7	8
9	10	11	12	13	14	15
16	17	18	19	20	21	22
23/30	24/31	25	26	27	28	29

april
s	m	t	w	t	f	s
		1	2	3	4	5
6	7	8	9	10	11	12
13	14	15	16	17	18	19
20	21	22	23	24	25	26
27	28	29	30			

may
s	m	t	w	t	f	s
				1	2	3
4	5	6	7	8	9	10
11	12	13	14	15	16	17
18	19	20	21	22	23	24
25	26	27	28	29	30	31

june
s	m	t	w	t	f	s
1	2	3	4	5	6	7
8	9	10	11	12	13	14
15	16	17	18	19	20	21
22	23	24	25	26	27	28
29	30					

july
s	m	t	w	t	f	s
		1	2	3	4	5
6	7	8	9	10	11	12
13	14	15	16	17	18	19
20	21	22	23	24	25	26
27	28	29	30	31		

august
s	m	t	w	t	f	s
					1	2
3	4	5	6	7	8	9
10	11	12	13	14	15	16
17	18	19	20	21	22	23
24/31	25	26	27	28	29	30

september
s	m	t	w	t	f	s
	1	2	3	4	5	6
7	8	9	10	11	12	13
14	15	16	17	18	19	20
21	22	23	24	25	26	27
28	29	30				

october
s	m	t	w	t	f	s
			1	2	3	4
5	6	7	8	9	10	11
12	13	14	15	16	17	18
19	20	21	22	23	24	25
26	27	28	29	30	31	

november
s	m	t	w	t	f	s
						1
2	3	4	5	6	7	8
9	10	11	12	13	14	15
16	17	18	19	20	21	22
23/30	24	25	26	27	28	29

december
s	m	t	w	t	f	s
	1	2	3	4	5	6
7	8	9	10	11	12	13
14	15	16	17	18	19	20
21	22	23	24	25	26	27
28	29	30	31			

1996

january
s	m	t	w	t	f	s
	1	2	3	4	5	6
7	8	9	10	11	12	13
14	15	16	17	18	19	20
21	22	23	24	25	26	27
28	29	30	31			

february
s	m	t	w	t	f	s
				1	2	3
4	5	6	7	8	9	10
11	12	13	14	15	16	17
18	19	20	21	22	23	24
25	26	27	28	29		

march
s	m	t	w	t	f	s
					1	2
3	4	5	6	7	8	9
10	11	12	13	14	15	16
17	18	19	20	21	22	23
24/31	25	26	27	28	29	30

april
s	m	t	w	t	f	s
	1	2	3	4	5	6
7	8	9	10	11	12	13
14	15	16	17	18	19	20
21	22	23	24	25	26	27
28	29	30				

may
s	m	t	w	t	f	s
			1	2	3	4
5	6	7	8	9	10	11
12	13	14	15	16	17	18
19	20	21	22	23	24	25
26	27	28	29	30	31	

june
s	m	t	w	t	f	s
						1
2	3	4	5	6	7	8
9	10	11	12	13	14	15
16	17	18	19	20	21	22
23/30	24	25	26	27	28	29

july
s	m	t	w	t	f	s
	1	2	3	4	5	6
7	8	9	10	11	12	13
14	15	16	17	18	19	20
21	22	23	24	25	26	27
28	29	30	31			

august
s	m	t	w	t	f	s
				1	2	3
4	5	6	7	8	9	10
11	12	13	14	15	16	17
18	19	20	21	22	23	24
25	26	27	28	29	30	31

september
s	m	t	w	t	f	s
1	2	3	4	5	6	7
8	9	10	11	12	13	14
15	16	17	18	19	20	21
22	23	24	25	26	27	28
29	30					

october
s	m	t	w	t	f	s
		1	2	3	4	5
6	7	8	9	10	11	12
13	14	15	16	17	18	19
20	21	22	23	24	25	26
27	28	29	30	31		

november
s	m	t	w	t	f	s
					1	2
3	4	5	6	7	8	9
10	11	12	13	14	15	16
17	18	19	20	21	22	23
24	25	26	27	28	29	30

december
s	m	t	w	t	f	s
1	2	3	4	5	6	7
8	9	10	11	12	13	14
15	16	17	18	19	20	21
22	23	24	25	26	27	28
29	30	31				

1998

january
s	m	t	w	t	f	s
				1	2	3
4	5	6	7	8	9	10
11	12	13	14	15	16	17
18	19	20	21	22	23	24
25	26	27	28	29	30	31

february
s	m	t	w	t	f	s
1	2	3	4	5	6	7
8	9	10	11	12	13	14
15	16	17	18	19	20	21
22	23	24	25	26	27	28

march
s	m	t	w	t	f	s
1	2	3	4	5	6	7
8	9	10	11	12	13	14
15	16	17	18	19	20	21
22	23	24	25	26	27	28
29	30	31				

april
s	m	t	w	t	f	s
			1	2	3	4
5	6	7	8	9	10	11
12	13	14	15	16	17	18
19	20	21	22	23	24	25
26	27	28	29	30		

may
s	m	t	w	t	f	s
					1	2
3	4	5	6	7	8	9
10	11	12	13	14	15	16
17	18	19	20	21	22	23
24/31	25	26	27	28	29	30

june
s	m	t	w	t	f	s
	1	2	3	4	5	6
7	8	9	10	11	12	13
14	15	16	17	18	19	20
21	22	23	24	25	26	27
28	29	30				

july
s	m	t	w	t	f	s
			1	2	3	4
5	6	7	8	9	10	11
12	13	14	15	16	17	18
19	20	21	22	23	24	25
26	27	28	29	30	31	

august
s	m	t	w	t	f	s
						1
2	3	4	5	6	7	8
9	10	11	12	13	14	15
16	17	18	19	20	21	22
23/30	24/31	25	26	27	28	29

september
s	m	t	w	t	f	s
		1	2	3	4	5
6	7	8	9	10	11	12
13	14	15	16	17	18	19
20	21	22	23	24	25	26
27	28	29	30			

october
s	m	t	w	t	f	s
				1	2	3
4	5	6	7	8	9	10
11	12	13	14	15	16	17
18	19	20	21	22	23	24
25	26	27	28	29	30	31

november
s	m	t	w	t	f	s
1	2	3	4	5	6	7
8	9	10	11	12	13	14
15	16	17	18	19	20	21
22	23	24	25	26	27	28
29	30					

december
s	m	t	w	t	f	s
		1	2	3	4	5
6	7	8	9	10	11	12
13	14	15	16	17	18	19
20	21	22	23	24	25	26
27	28	29	30	31		

1999

january
s	m	t	w	t	f	s
					1	2
3	4	5	6	7	8	9
10	11	12	13	14	15	16
17	18	19	20	21	22	23
24/31	25	26	27	28	29	30

february
s	m	t	w	t	f	s
	1	2	3	4	5	6
7	8	9	10	11	12	13
14	15	16	17	18	19	20
21	22	23	24	25	26	27
28						

march
s	m	t	w	t	f	s
	1	2	3	4	5	6
7	8	9	10	11	12	13
14	15	16	17	18	19	20
21	22	23	24	25	26	27
28	29	30	31			

april
s	m	t	w	t	f	s
				1	2	3
4	5	6	7	8	9	10
11	12	13	14	15	16	17
18	19	20	21	22	23	24
25	26	27	28	29	30	

may
s	m	t	w	t	f	s
						1
2	3	4	5	6	7	8
9	10	11	12	13	14	15
16	17	18	19	20	21	22
23/30	24/31	25	26	27	28	29

june
s	m	t	w	t	f	s
		1	2	3	4	5
6	7	8	9	10	11	12
13	14	15	16	17	18	19
20	21	22	23	24	25	26
27	28	29	30			

july
s	m	t	w	t	f	s
				1	2	3
4	5	6	7	8	9	10
11	12	13	14	15	16	17
18	19	20	21	22	23	24
25	26	27	28	29	30	31

august
s	m	t	w	t	f	s
1	2	3	4	5	6	7
8	9	10	11	12	13	14
15	16	17	18	19	20	21
22	23	24	25	26	27	28
29	30	31				

september
s	m	t	w	t	f	s
			1	2	3	4
5	6	7	8	9	10	11
12	13	14	15	16	17	18
19	20	21	22	23	24	25
26	27	28	29	30		

october
s	m	t	w	t	f	s
					1	2
3	4	5	6	7	8	9
10	11	12	13	14	15	16
17	18	19	20	21	22	23
24/31	25	26	27	28	29	30

november
s	m	t	w	t	f	s
	1	2	3	4	5	6
7	8	9	10	11	12	13
14	15	16	17	18	19	20
21	22	23	24	25	26	27
28	29	30				

december
s	m	t	w	t	f	s
			1	2	3	4
5	6	7	8	9	10	11
12	13	14	15	16	17	18
19	20	21	22	23	24	25
26	27	28	29	30	31	

HOLIDAYS

january 1, wednesday . . . . . new year's day
january 20, monday
    martin luther king, jr. birthday celebration
february 12, wednesday . . lincoln's birthday
february 12, wednesday . . . . . ash wednesday
february 14, friday . . . . . valentine's day
february 17, monday . . . . . presidents' day
february 22, saturday . washington's birthday
march 17, monday . . . . . . st. patrick's day
march 23, sunday . . . . palm sunday
march 28, friday . . . . good friday
march 30, sunday . . . . easter
march 31, monday . . . easter monday (canada)
april 22, tuesday . . . . . . passover begins
may 11, sunday . . . . mother's day
may 19, monday . . . . victoria day (canada)
may 26, monday . . . . memorial day
june 14, saturday . . . . flag day

june 15, sunday . . . . father's day
june 24, tuesday . . . .
                    st. jean-baptiste day (canada)
july 1, tuesday . . . . . . canada day (canada)
july 4, friday . . . . independence day
september 1, monday . . . . labor day
october 2, thursday . . . . . rosh hashanah
october 11, saturday . . . . yom kippur
october 13, monday . . . . columbus day
october 13, monday . . . thanksgiving (canada)
october 31, friday . . . . halloween
november 4, tuesday . . . . . . election day
november 11, tuesday . . . . . . veterans day
november 11, tuesday remembrance day (canada)
november 27, thursday thanksgiving day (u.s.)
december 24, wednesday . . . . hanukkah begins
december 25, thursday . . . . christmas
december 26, friday . . . boxing day (canada)

The airplane passenger manifest that Scully scrutinizes in "Little Green Men" while trying to trace Mulder's movements, contains the names of many online X-Files fans.

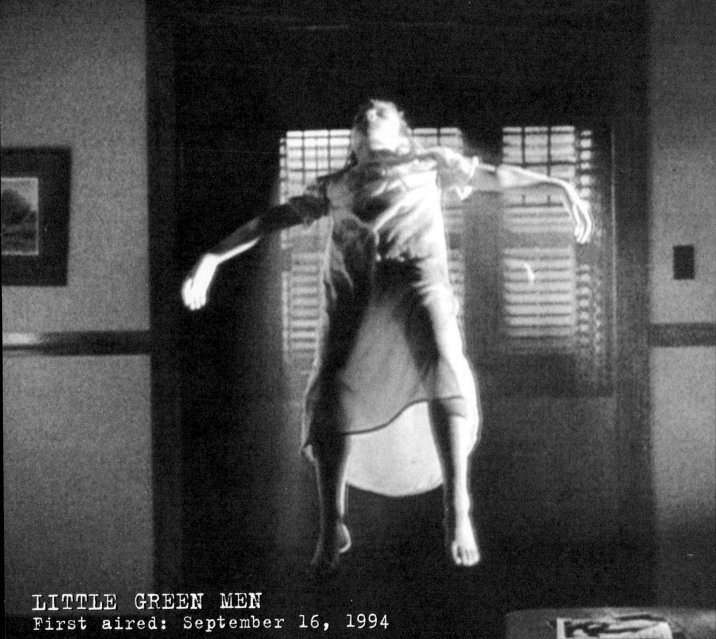

LITTLE GREEN MEN
First aired: September 16, 1994

DECEMBER/JANUARY

30 monday

31 tuesday

1 wednesday (new year's day)

2 thursday

3 friday

4 saturday

5 sunday

X

In January 1994, The X-Files won the Golden Globe Award for Best Dramatic Series.

JANUARY

6 monday

7 tuesday

8 wednesday

9 thursday

10 friday

_____
_____
_____
_____
_____
_____

11 saturday

_____
_____
_____
_____
_____

12 sunday

_____
_____
_____
_____
_____

X

January 7, 1948. Captain Thomas
Mantell of the U.S. Air Force
pursued a UFO he described as
"metallic and tremendous in
size;" his body and crashed
plane were later found after
he lost contact with ground
control.

JANUARY

13 monday _____

_____

_____

_____

_____

_____

14 tuesday _____

_____

_____

_____

_____

_____

15 wednesday _____

_____

_____

_____

_____

_____

16 thursday _____

_____

_____

_____

_____

_____

17 friday

18 saturday

19 sunday

X

A rare alignment of the planets, which occurs on January 12, 1996, plunges Mulder and Scully into a town swept up by strange behavior and murderous teens. "SYZYGY"

JANUARY

20 monday (martin luther king, jr. birthday celebration)

21 tuesday

22 wednesday

23 thursday

24 friday

_____
_____
_____
_____
_____
_____

25 saturday

_____
_____
_____
_____
_____

26 sunday

_____
_____
_____
_____
_____
_____
_____

X

Mulder and Scully investigate
the case of a gender-switching
killer who murders his victims
through sex. "GENDERBENDER"

JANUARY/FEBRUARY

27 monday

28 tuesday

29 wednesday

30 thursday

31 friday

1 saturday

2 sunday

X

In a New Hampshire woods a young boy summoning a demon to impress his date calls up more than he can handle.
"DIE HAND DIE VERLETZT"

The aristocratic British lord, Sir Malcolm Marsden, who is threatened by a pyrokinetic assassin in "Fire," was actually named after the show's chief hairdresser.

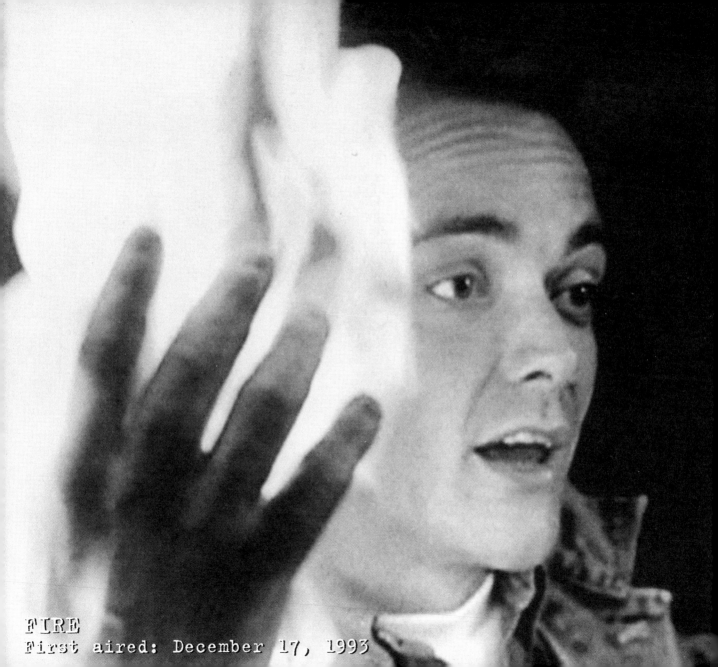

FIRE
First aired: December 17, 1993

FEBRUARY

3 monday

4 tuesday

5 wednesday

6 thursday

7 friday

8 saturday

9 sunday

X

February 3, 1995. Agent Mulder
arrives in the Arctic Circle
searching for the alien assassin
who killed a clone claiming to
be his sister.
"END GAME"

FEBRUARY

10 monday _____   **11 tuesday** _____

_____   _____

_____   _____

_____   _____

_____   _____

_____   _____

_____   _____

12 wednesday (lincoln's birthday)   **13 thursday** _____
(ash wednesday)

_____   _____

_____   _____

_____   _____

_____   _____

_____   _____

14 friday (valentine's day)

15 saturday

Today was a special day. Today was the day I met Brenda. I wounder what is going to transpire between the two of us.

16 sunday

X

Mulder's old nemesis, John Barnett, kills a jewelry store clerk just to send Mulder a message—that he's not dead. "YOUNG AT HEART"

FEBRUARY

17 monday (presidents' day)

18 tuesday

19 wednesday

20 thursday

21 friday

_____
_____
_____
_____
_____
_____

22 saturday

_____
_____
_____
_____
_____

23 sunday

_____
_____
_____
_____
_____
_____

X

An Iraqi fighter pilot shoots
down a UFO, and Deep Throat leads
Mulder on a merry chase across
the country looking for it.
"E.B.E."

FEBRUARY/MARCH

24 monday

25 tuesday

26 wednesday

27 thursday

28 friday _____   1 saturday *Nana's B-Day* _____

_____   _____

_____   _____

_____   _____

_____   _____

_____   _____

_____   _____

2 sunday _____

_____   # X

_____   Dana Scully was born February 23,
                                 1964.
_____

_____

_____

_____

The final episode of season one, "The Erlenmeyer Flask," marks the departure from the series of Deep Throat (played by Jerry Hardin), the undercover source for Mulder. His dying words, "Trust no one," are substituted in the teaser for the show's usual "The truth is out there."

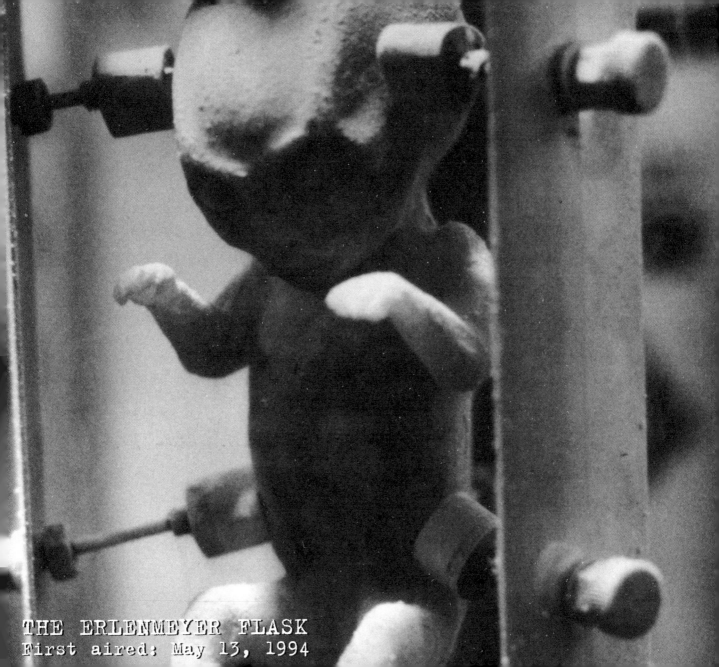

THE ERLENMEYER FLASK
First aired: May 13, 1994

MARCH

3 monday

4 tuesday

5 wednesday

6 thursday

Michelle Whall's B-Day

7 friday

8 saturday

9 sunday

X

March 6, 1992. Dana Scully is
assigned to the X-Files division
and meets Fox Mulder.
THE X-FILES PILOT

MARCH

10 monday *My B-Day*

I took Brenda out for my
Birthday. We went to the
Weather vane.

11 tuesday

Took Brenda to Therapy.

12 wednesday

Took Brenda to see doctor.
Saw inside of Spencer Press.

13 thursday

14 friday

_____
_____
_____
_____
_____
_____

15 saturday

_____
_____
_____
_____
_____
_____

16 sunday

_____
_____
_____
_____
_____
_____
_____

X

March 9, 1993. Samuel Hartley
rises from a slab at the
morgue to face down a killer
from his own congregation.
"MIRACLE MAN"

MARCH

17 monday (st. patrick's day)

18 tuesday

19 wednesday

20 thursday

21 friday

_____
_____
_____
_____
_____
_____

22 saturday

_____
_____
_____
_____
_____

23 sunday (palm sunday)

_____
_____
_____
_____
_____
_____
_____

X

Mulder and Scully close their
first case together on March 22,
1992 by subjecting Billy Miles
to hypnotic regression; Miles
claims to have been abducted and
to have had implants inserted in
his sinuses.
THE X-FILES PILOT

MARCH

<u>24 monday</u>

<u>25 tuesday</u>

<u>26 wednesday</u>

<u>27 thursday</u>

28 friday (good friday)

_____
_____
_____
_____
_____
_____

29 saturday

_____
_____
_____
_____
_____
_____

30 sunday (easter)

_____
_____
_____
_____
_____
_____

X

March 27, 1994. Mulder and
Scully open the file on
Michelle Bishop, a little girl
who may house the soul of a
murdered cop. "BORN AGAIN"

The bones and skulls used in "Aubrey" are not real bones. They are plastic bones which must be "aged" with paint and chemicals, and have the plastic seams filed off. Real bones would cost a great deal more.

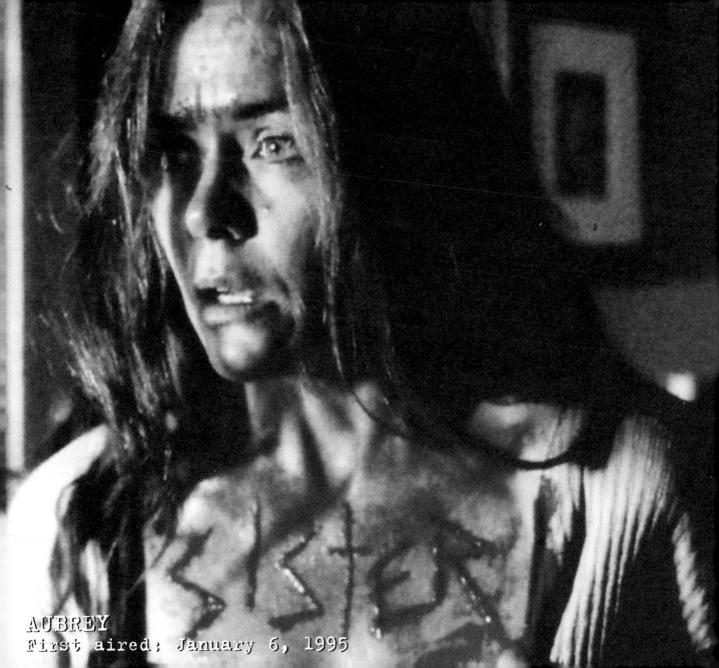

AUBREY
First aired: January 6, 1995

MARCH/APRIL

31 monday (easter monday-canada)
_____
_____
_____
_____
_____
_____

1 tuesday
_____
_____
_____
_____
_____
_____

2 wednesday
_____
_____
_____
_____
_____
_____

3 thursday
_____
_____
_____
_____
_____
_____

4 friday

5 saturday

6 sunday   (daylight saving time begins)

X
_____

A bizarre murder in a circus town draws Mulder and Scully into an investigation involving sideshow freaks and geeks. "HUMBUG"

APRIL

7 monday

8 tuesday

9 wednesday

10 thursday

11 friday

12 saturday

13 sunday

X

April 9, 1995. An earthquake on a Navajo reservation in Arizona uncovers a buried box-car full of what appear to be alien bodies.
"ANASAZI"

APRIL

14 monday _____

15 tuesday _____

16 wednesday *Mom B-Day*

17 thursday _____

18 friday _____

19 saturday _____

_____

_____

_____

_____

_____

20 sunday _____

_____

_____

_____

_____

X
___

April 16, 1995. "The Thinker"
is found murdered in a Trenton
dump site, alerting Scully to
Fox Mulder's frame-up for his
father's murder. "BLESSING WAY"

APRIL

21 monday _____

22 tuesday (passover begins) _____

23 wednesday _____

24 thursday _____

<u>25 friday</u>

<u>26 saturday</u>

<u>27 sunday</u>

X

April 25, 1994. Mentally
retarded janitor Roland Fuller,
under the psychic control of
his dead twin, kills a scien-
tist by holding his head in a
vat of liquid nitrogen.
"ROLAND"

APRIL/MAY

28 monday

29 tuesday

30 wednesday

1 thursday

2 friday _____

3 saturday _____

4 sunday _____

X

May 2, 1993. Lula Phillips,
released from prison, begins a
crime spree with Warren Dupre.
"LAZARUS"

The Flukeman costume in "The Host" was a true ordeal for actor Darin Morgan. Originally it took six hours to put on before technicians were able to speed up the process, and at one point in the filming Morgan had to wear the costume for 20 consecutive hours.

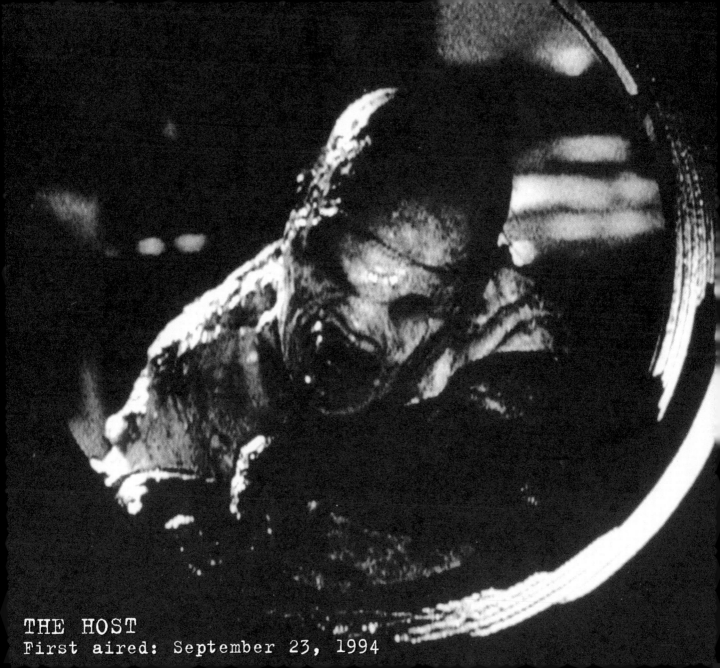

THE HOST
First aired: September 23, 1994

5 monday

6 tuesday

7 wednesday

8 thursday

9 friday

_____

_____

_____

_____

_____

10 saturday

_____

_____

_____

_____

_____

11 sunday (mother's day)

_____

_____

_____

_____

_____

_____

X

May 8, 1994. Dr. Secare, a man cured of cancer by alien gene therapy, is shot by Baltimore police and bleeds green blood. "THE ERLENMEYER FLASK"

MAY

12 monday

13 tuesday

14 wednesday

15 thursday

16 friday

_____
_____
_____
_____
_____
_____

17 saturday

_____
_____
_____
_____
_____

18 sunday

_____
_____
_____
_____
_____
_____

X

George Kearns meets a grisly
end at the hands of cannibals
in the small town of Dudley,
Arkansas. "OUR TOWN"

MAY

19 monday (victoria day-canada)

20 tuesday

21 wednesday

22 thursday

23 friday

24 saturday

25 sunday

X

Under the influence of a drug planted in his tap water, Mulder hits Skinner in the face. "ANASAZI"

MAY/JUNE

26 monday (memorial day)

27 tuesday

28 wednesday

29 thursday

30 friday

_____
_____
_____
_____
_____
_____

31 saturday

_____
_____
_____
_____
_____

1 sunday

_____
_____
_____
_____
_____
_____

X

May 26, 1994. Assistant
Director Walter Skinner, acting
on orders, closes the X-Files
and re-assigns Mulder and
Scully to other duties.
"THE ERLENMEYER FLASK"

Mulder tells Roland a dream he (Mulder) had, wherein he dove down into a pool searching for his father. In the script, Mulder was searching for his sister.

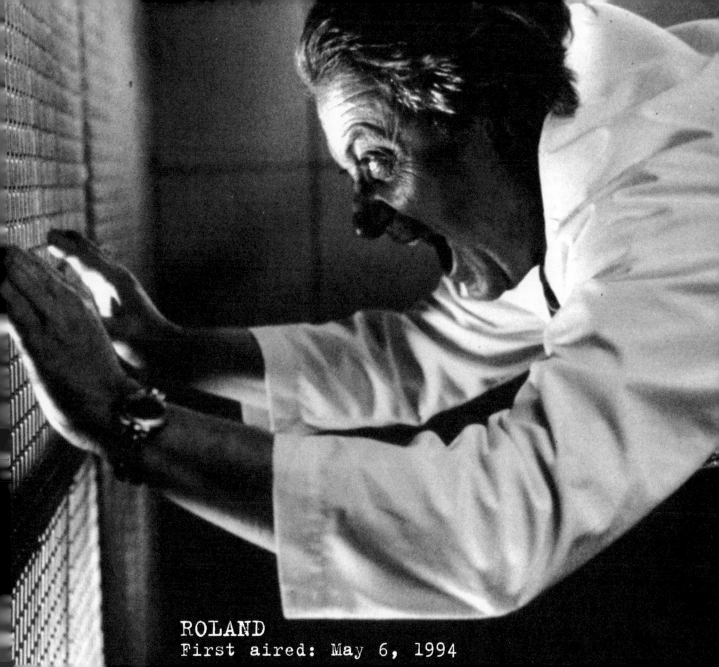

ROLAND
First aired: May 6, 1994

JUNE

2 monday
_____
_____
_____
_____
_____
_____
_____

3 tuesday
_____
_____
_____
_____
_____
_____
_____

4 wednesday
_____
_____
_____
_____
_____
_____
_____

5 thursday
_____
_____
_____
_____
_____
_____
_____

6 friday

_____
_____
_____
_____
_____
_____

7 saturday

_____
_____
_____
_____
_____

8 sunday

_____
_____
_____
_____
_____
_____

X
___

June 3, 1985. Duane Barry is
abducted from his home in
Pulaski, Virginia. "DUANE BARRY"

JUNE

9 monday

10 tuesday *Lee R-Day*

11 wednesday

12 thursday

13 friday

_____
_____
_____
_____
_____
_____

14 saturday (flag day)

_____
_____
_____
_____
_____
_____

15 sunday (father's day)

_____
_____
_____
_____
_____
_____

X

The football game that Mulder and Scully miss in order to investigate a grisly serial killer is Washington v. Minnesota, two teams that each had a "Carter" in their ranks. In one scene a television announcer mentions a catch by Cris Carter. "IRRESISTIBLE"

JUNE

16 monday

17 tuesday

18 wednesday

19 thursday

20 friday

21 saturday

22 sunday

X

June 16, 1989. Fox Mulder
undergoes hypnotic regression
with Dr. Heitz Verber and
recovers memories of his sister's abduction. "CONDUIT"

JUNE

23 monday

24 tuesday (st. jean-baptiste day-
canada)

25 wednesday

26 thursday

27 friday

_____
_____
_____
_____
_____
_____

28 saturday

_____
_____
_____
_____
_____

29 sunday

_____
_____
_____
_____
_____

X

June 24, 1947. Kenneth Arnold's historic sighting of disks flying over the Cascade Mountains gave rise to the phrase "flying saucers," the first use of the term in UFO literature.

The concept for "Dod Kalm" was built around access the X-Files crew had to a Canadian navy destroyer. The writers were specifically asked to tailor a script around that setting.

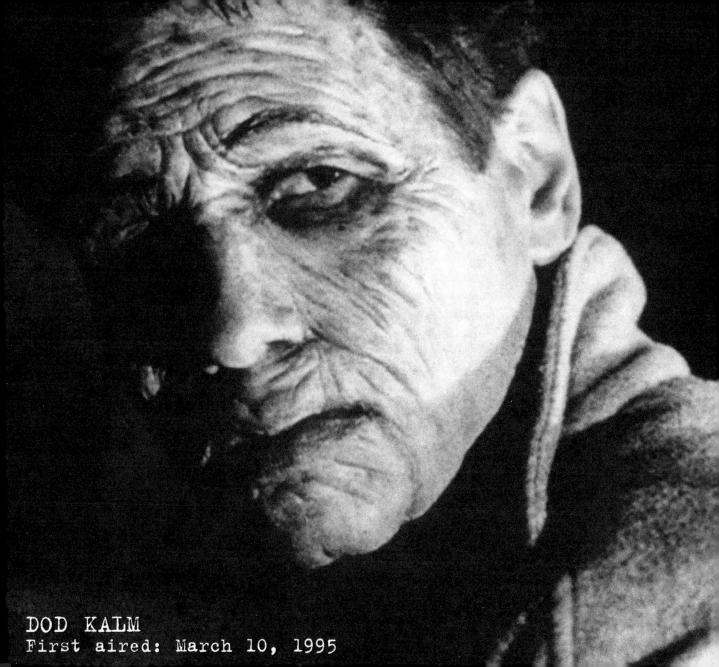

DOD KALM
First aired: March 10, 1995

JUNE/JULY

30 monday

1 tuesday (canada day-canada)

2 wednesday

3 thursday

4 friday   (independence day)

_____
_____
_____
_____
_____
_____

5 saturday   Dad B-Day

_____
_____
_____
_____
_____
_____

6 sunday

_____
_____
_____
_____
_____
_____
_____

X

July 2, 1947 Witnesses claimed to
have found a crashed UFO on a
ranch outside Roswell, NM.
Although government reports
initially labeled it a "flying
disk," later reports claimed that
it was a weather balloon.

JULY

7 monday

8 tuesday

9 wednesday

10 thursday

11 friday

12 saturday

13 sunday

X

July 7, 1994. Mulder flies to Puerto Rico to investigate the possibility of extraterrestrial contact. "LITTLE GREEN MEN"

14 monday

15 tuesday

16 wednesday

17 thursday

18 friday

19 saturday

20 sunday

X

Chris Carter has appeared on
The X-Files only once: he was
one of the FBI panel members
interviewing Scully in the
episode "ANASAZI."

JULY

21 monday

22 tuesday

23 wednesday

24 thursday

25 friday

_____
_____
_____
_____
_____
_____

26 saturday

_____
_____
_____
_____
_____
_____

27 sunday

_____
_____
_____
_____
_____
_____

X
_____

July 23, 1993. Eugene Victor
Tooms is arrested for tearing
the liver out of George
Usher, but is released after
he passes a lie detector test.
"SQUEEZE"

28 monday

29 tuesday

30 wednesday

31 thursday

1 friday

2 saturday

3 sunday

X

Senator Richard Matheson, who
sends Mulder to Arecibo,
Puerto Rico, is named for
science fiction and horror
writer Richard "Somewhere in
Time" Matheson.

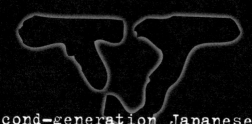

Nisei: Second-generation Japanese-Americans.
In the episode by that title the term refers
to the subjects of experiments conducted by a
Japanese war criminal in the United States.

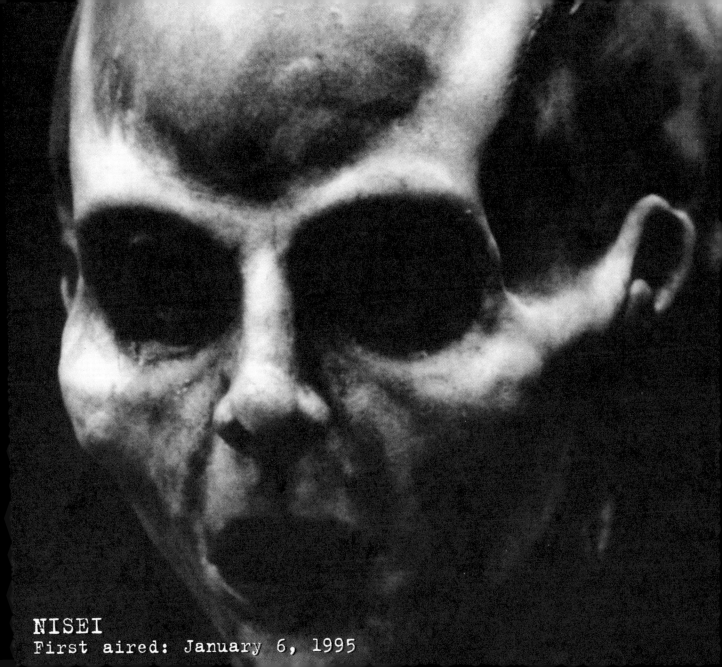

NISEI
First aired: January 6, 1995

AUGUST

4 monday

5 tuesday

6 wednesday

7 thursday

8 friday *Dave'n B-Day*

9 saturday

10 sunday

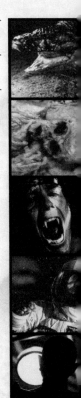

X

David Duchovny born August 7, 1960.

Gillian Anderson born August 9, 1968.

AUGUST

11 monday

12 tuesday

13 wednesday

14 thursday

15 friday

_____
_____
_____
_____
_____

16 saturday

_____
_____
_____
_____
_____

17 sunday

_____
_____
_____
_____
_____

X

August 10, 1944. On a bomber mission over India, Capt. A. M. Reida sighted "foo fighters" following his craft. He described spheres "five or six feet in diameter, bright orange" which paced his plane at 210 mph.

AUGUST

18 monday

19 tuesday

20 wednesday

21 thursday

22 friday

23 saturday

24 sunday

X

August 19, 1953. A sailor
dying of radiation burns tells
Bill Mulder and the young
Cigarette-Smoking Man of his
submarine's suicide mission to
guard a sunken UFO. "APOCRYPHA"

AUGUST

25 monday
_____
_____
_____
_____
_____
_____

26 tuesday
_____
_____
_____
_____
_____
_____

27 wednesday
_____
_____
_____
_____
_____
_____

28 thursday
_____
_____
_____
_____
_____
_____

29 friday _____

30 saturday _____

31 sunday _____

X

August 29, 1995. Dana Scully
attempts to autopsy the remains
of Lauren MacKalvey and finds
most of the fatty tissue miss-
ing from her corpse. "2 SHY"

The case of Phineas Gage, which Scully refers
to in "Duane Barry," actually happened.
In the early part of this century, a railway worker
placing dynamite set off an explosion that drove a
three-foot-long steel rod through his brain. Gage
not only survived but suffered no physical
impairment and went on to live another 20
years. However, his personality underwent a
dramatic change, turning him into an irascible,
profane, and thoroughly unpleasant man.

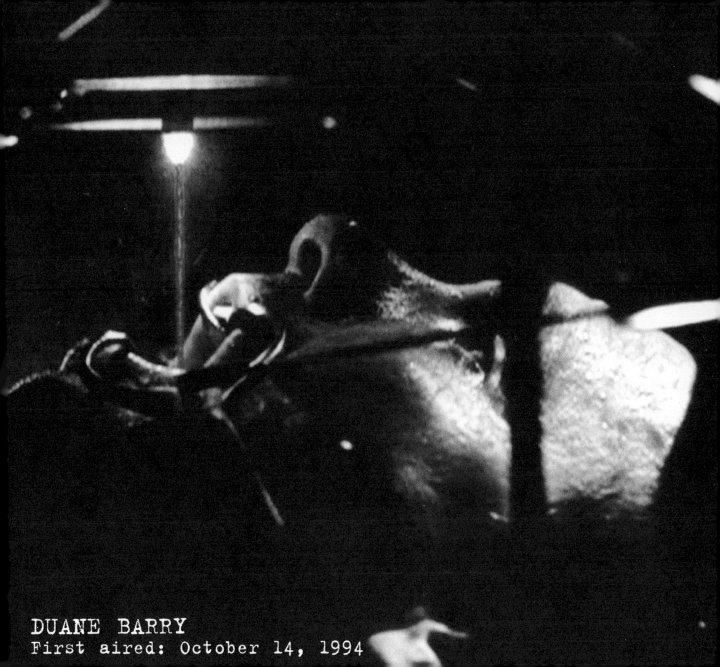

DUANE BARRY
First aired: October 14, 1994

SEPTEMBER

1 monday (labor day)

2 tuesday

3 wednesday

4 thursday

5 friday

6 saturday

7 sunday

X

"Crowley" High School evokes
the memory of British ceremoni-
alist Aleister Crowley, whose
theories on "magick" shocked
his contemporaries and heavily
influenced the development of
modern Wicca.
"DIE HAND DIE VERLETZT"

SEPTEMBER

8 monday

9 tuesday

10 wednesday

11 thursday

12 friday _____

_____

_____

_____

_____

_____

13 saturday _____

_____

_____

_____

_____

14 sunday _____

_____

_____

_____

_____

X

September 12, 1995. Darren
Peter Oswald sets a new record
on a video game after killing
a pizza delivery boy with a
lightning bolt. "D.P.O."

SEPTEMBER

15 monday

_____
_____
_____
_____
_____
_____

16 tuesday

_____
_____
_____
_____
_____
_____

17 wednesday

_____
_____
_____
_____
_____
_____

18 thursday

_____
_____
_____
_____
_____
_____

19 friday

_____

_____

_____

_____

_____

20 saturday

_____

_____

_____

_____

_____

21 sunday

_____

_____

_____

_____

_____

_____

X
—

September 16, 1995. Clyde
Bruckman finds the body of a
murdered fortune-teller; Mulder
discovers Bruckman is psychic.
"CLYDE BRUCKMAN'S FINAL REPOSE"

SEPTEMBER

22 monday

23 tuesday

24 wednesday

25 thursday

26 friday

27 saturday

28 sunday

X

Piper Maru Anderson, Gillian
Anderson's daughter, born
September 25, 1994.

Deep Throat's warning in the "Fallen Angel" episode is a quote from Don Corleone in The Godfather. "Keep your friends close, but keep your enemies closer."

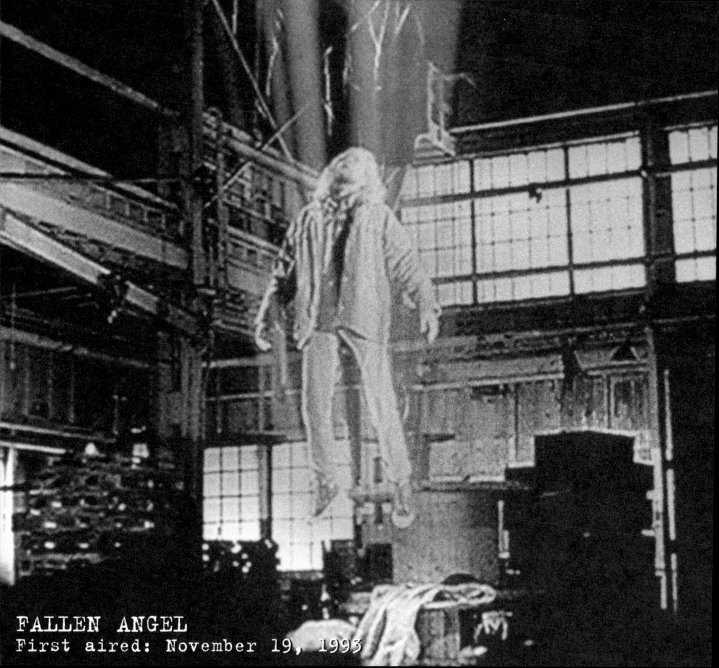

FALLEN ANGEL
First aired: November 19, 1993

SEPTEMBER/OCTOBER

29 monday

30 tuesday

1 wednesday

2 thursday (rosh hashanah)

3 friday

_____

_____

_____

_____

_____

_____

4 saturday

_____

_____

_____

_____

_____

_____

5 sunday

_____

_____

_____

_____

_____

_____

X

October 1, 1993. Mulder and
Scully investigate the abduction of a young girl, prompt-
ing Mulder to confront his
feelings about his own sister's
disappearance. "CONDUIT"

OCTOBER

6 monday
_____
_____
_____
_____
_____
_____

7 tuesday
_____
_____
_____
_____
_____
_____

8 wednesday
_____
_____
_____
_____
_____

9 thursday
_____
_____
_____
_____
_____

10 friday

11 saturday (yom kippur)

12 sunday

X

October 5, 1993. Howard
Graves is murdered and his
death made to look like suicide; his ghost returns to
protect his secretary.
"SHADOWS"

OCTOBER

13 monday (columbus day)
(thanksgiving-canada)

14 tuesday

15 wednesday

16 thursday

17 friday

_____
_____
_____
_____
_____
_____

18 saturday

_____
_____
_____
_____
_____
_____

19 sunday

_____
_____
_____
_____
_____
_____

X
___

Fox Mulder born October 13, 1961.
Series creator Chris Carter
born October 13, 1956. "Ten
Thirteen Productions" is named
for his birthday.

OCTOBER

20 monday

21 tuesday

22 wednesday

23 thursday

24 friday

25 saturday

26 sunday (daylight saving time ends)

X

October 24, 1993. Mulder and
Scully investigate the locked-
room murder of a man; suspicion
falls on a self-aware computer
of murderous intent.
"GHOST IN THE MACHINE"

27 monday

28 tuesday

29 wednesday

30 thursday

31 friday (halloween)

1 saturday

2 sunday

X

October 27, 1995. Virgil Incanto's skin, found at the scene of one of his crimes, reveals his unusual disorder and sends Mulder and Scully looking for a "fat-sucking vampire." "2 SHY"

The design which appears on a tree in the beginning of "Fresh Bones" is a "vever," a sign belonging to the spirits honored in voudoun. As Bauvais explains, the vever is a loco-miroir, or mirror of the soul.

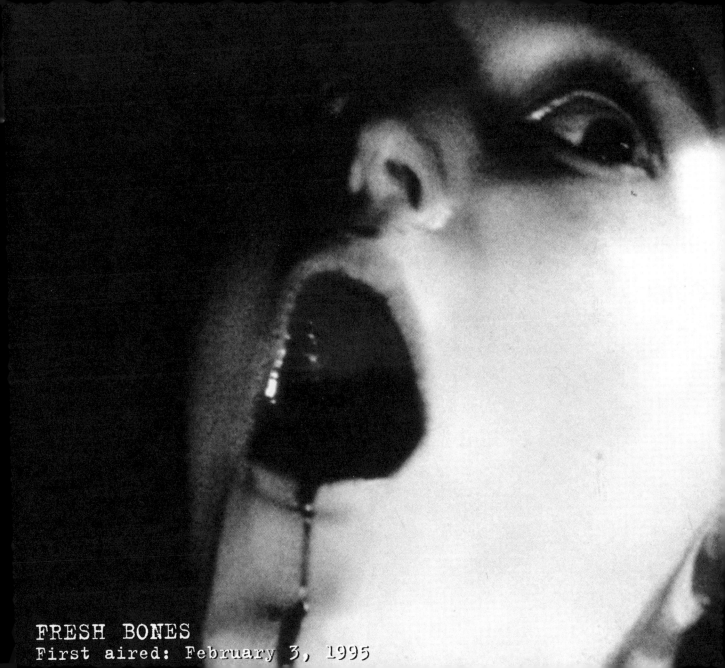

FRESH BONES
First aired: February 3, 1995

NOVEMBER

3 monday

4 tuesday (election day)

5 wednesday

6 thursday

7 friday

_____
_____
_____
_____
_____
_____

8 saturday

_____
_____
_____
_____
_____
_____

9 sunday

_____
_____
_____
_____
_____
_____

X

November 5, 1993. Mulder and
Scully investigate the deaths
of an entire Arctic research
crew and find themselves
trapped with an alien parasite.
"ICE"

NOVEMBER

10 monday

11 tuesday (veterans day) (remembrance day-canada)

12 wednesday

13 thursday

14 friday

15 saturday

16 sunday

X

November 14, 1994. Donnie Pfaster, arrested for assaulting a girl in his classroom, catches sight of Agent Scully and targets her for his next victim. "IRRESISTIBLE"

NOVEMBER

<u>17 monday</u>

_____

_____

_____

_____

_____

<u>18 tuesday</u>

_____

_____

_____

_____

_____

<u>19 wednesday</u>

_____

_____

_____

_____

_____

<u>20 thursday</u>

_____

_____

_____

_____

_____

21 friday _____

_____

_____

_____

_____

_____

22 saturday _____

_____

_____

_____

_____

_____

23 sunday _____

_____

_____

_____

_____

_____

_____

X

Samantha Mulder born November 21, 1965. "PAPER CLIP."

NOVEMBER

24 monday

25 tuesday

26 wednesday

27 thursday (thanksgiving day-u.s.)

28 friday

29 saturday

30 sunday

X

November 27, 1973. Agent Fox
Mulder's sister Samantha is
abducted from their home.
Mulder later remembers "a
presence in the room" and a
bright light, and believes she
was taken by aliens.
"LITTLE GREEN MEN"

"One Breath" was filmed just days after Gillian Anderson gave birth to her daughter Piper by cesarean section. Scully spends most of the episode lying in a hospital bed, unconscious, while Mulder fights to save her life.

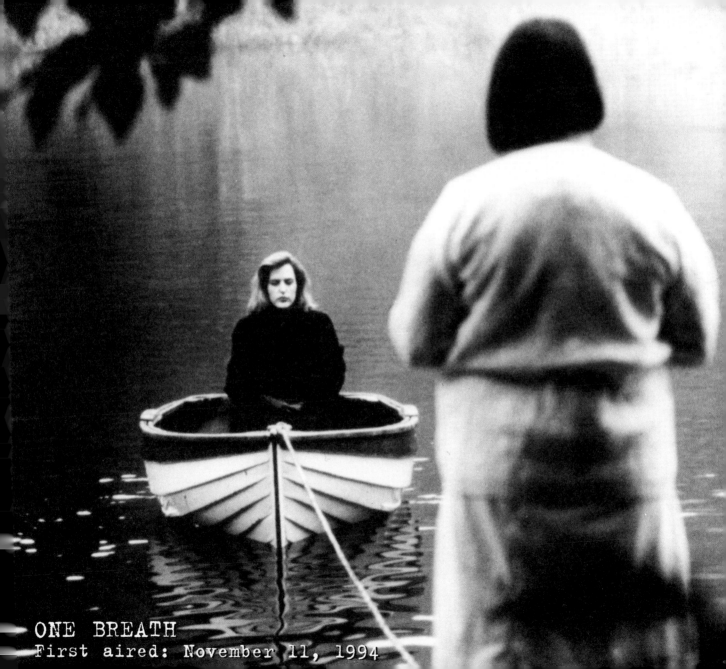
ONE BREATH
First aired: November 11, 1994

DECEMBER

1 monday
_____
_____
_____
_____
_____
_____

2 tuesday
_____
_____
_____
_____
_____
_____

3 wednesday
_____
_____
_____
_____
_____
_____

4 thursday
_____
_____
_____
_____
_____
_____

5 friday

6 saturday

7 sunday

X

"3" is the only episode to be
made without Gillian Anderson.

DECEMBER

8 monday

9 tuesday

10 wednesday

11 thursday

12 friday

_____
_____
_____
_____
_____

13 saturday

_____
_____
_____
_____
_____

14 sunday

_____
_____
_____
_____
_____

X
___

December 11, 1984. Los Angeles
TV producer Jaime Shandera
received the famous "Majestic
12" documents, purportedly
proving that the government
covered up the existence of
a UFO recovered from the
Roswell crash.

DECEMBER

15 monday

16 tuesday

17 wednesday

18 thursday

19 friday

20 saturday

21 sunday

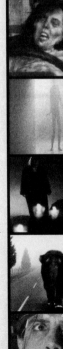

X

Scully and Mulder clash over
the causes of a stigmata in
young Kevin Cryder, even as a
diabolical killer stalks
the boy. "REVELATIONS"

DECEMBER

22 monday _____

23 tuesday _____

24 wednesday (hanukkah begins) _____

25 thursday (christmas) _____

26 friday (boxing day) canada

27 saturday

28 sunday

X

Captain William Scully, Agent Dana Scully's father, dies between Christmas 1993 and New Year's 1994. "BEYOND THE SEA"

DECEMBER/JANUARY

29 monday

30 tuesday

31 wednesday

1 thursday (new year's day)

2 friday _____

3 saturday _____

_____

_____

_____

_____

_____

4 sunday _____

X

December 29, 1994. "Dr.
Landon Prince," one of the
cloned Gregors, is killed by
an alien assassin sent to wipe
out the group's attempt to
hybridize humans and aliens.
"COLONY"

NOTES

_____
_____
_____
_____
_____
_____
_____
_____
_____
_____
_____
_____
_____
_____
_____
_____
_____

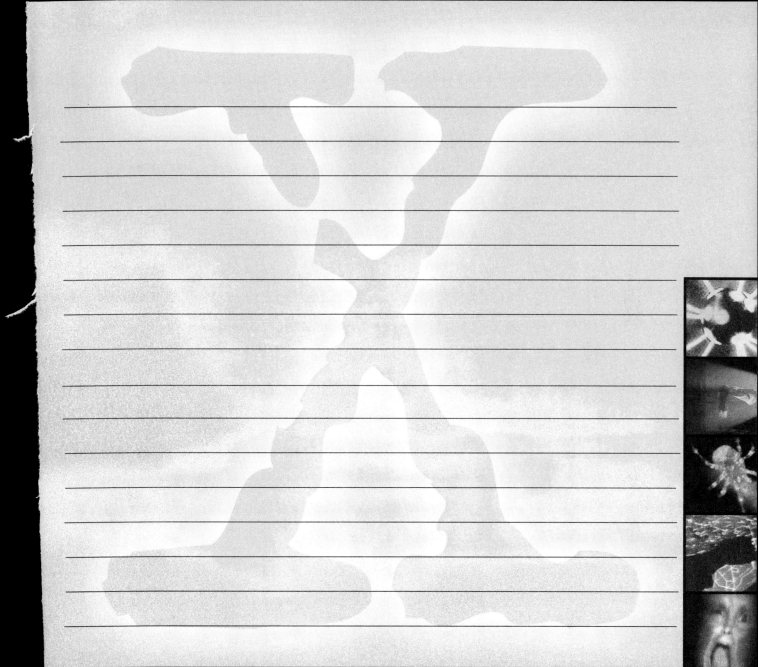

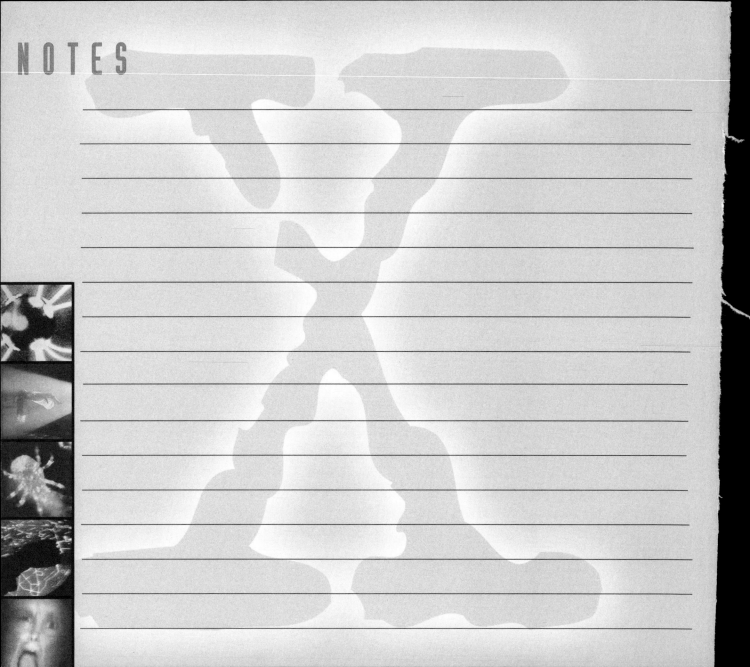